# 5:2 Diet

# Lose Weight Fast with the 5:2 Intermittent Fasting Diet

KARA AIMER

# CONTENTS

# INTRODUCTION

Going on a diet can be an extremely tough decision to make. The kind of diet you would choose really depends on how much weight you have to lose, how much movement you want to do and even on how much money you want to spend out of your pocket. Some diets can be costly as it would require you to buy expensive shakes or supplements. Fortunately, the 5:2 Diet is not of that kind – you won't need to spend hundreds of dollars each and every month just to achieve your goal of losing weight. and then keep on paying just to maintain it. This diet will show you how to lose the weight and keep it off for good at a fair price.

Before we get into the dieting aspect, here are some tips for starting your dieting routine:

Follow through with your eating plan: Taking a few days or a week off will completely reset your system and you will have to start over from day one. With this diet, that isn't advisable.

Start small: When you start on the 5:2 Diet plan, you might be making a significant calorie cut. So you might want to start by going down slowly instead of following the plan directly. Of course, once you get to the 5:2 Diet level, you shouldn't go backwards.

Be realistic: Even if you have a diet made just for you by a professional, you won't lose 20 pounds overnight. You have to be realistic about the amount of weight you want to lose and how much time you are giving yourself to lose it.

Reward yourself, don't punish yourself: One great tip that people use is to create a jar with pebbles in it. Each pebble represents a pound. When you see yourself losing weight, you transfer the pebbles from one jar to the other. Set reward levels for yourself: New shoes, new sunglasses, a movie or a vacation. Just make sure that your reward isn't going to be food!

Find a diet buddy: Research has shown that people who go on diets alone are not nearly as successful as those who do it with support. Find someone what will hold you accountable for your day-to-day actions. It doesn't matter if the buddy is someone in your family, your significant other, your friend or even someone online – just get someone who is rooting you on!

Eat clean foods: Make sure you learn how to read food labels. Be wary of foods that are low fat or low sodium – they often make that taste up somewhere else. When in doubt, eat as clean as possible and avoid processed foods.

Add in exercise: Diet is the key to losing weight, but exercise is also important. Start as slow as you want, with just twenty-minute walks, but you will eventually want to work yourself up to taking longer walks, jogging, adding weights or riding bicycles.

# WHAT IS THE 5:2 DIET?

The 5:2 Diet doesn't require you to purchase extra food, supplements, shakes or diet pills. Instead, it is all about you and your ability to restrict your calories two days a week. You will simply restrict your calorie consumption to only 25% of what you need in a day. You will do this two days a week (three if you need to lose weight quickly, and one day a week to maintain weight loss) while eating normally every other day of the week. You will be consuming fewer calories than you normally need, but you also aren't putting your body into starvation mode. Starvation mode occurs when your body does not receive the nutrition that it needs to fulfill day-to-day activities. It often occurs when you don't eat the calories you need for several days in a row. By regularly eating most of the time and having two days that you don't eat as much, especially if they are not next to each other, you won't go into starvation mode.

In addition to weight loss and generally feeling better, there are other health benefits as well. The real name for what you are doing is intermittent fasting – it is used in a variety of diets. Intermittent fasting acts to help your body repair its cells and cell walls, which will help your body stay healthy and fight off diseases like heart diseases, stroke, Alzheimer's and other forms of dementia, type 2 diabetes and cancer.

After just a few weeks on the 5:2 Diet, people of all sizes, genders, and backgrounds have reported that they had improved test results when it came to blood pressure and cholesterol testing. This testing was even better after months, coupled with the diet type and the significant weight loss. People, who were unable to lose weight before, have lost enough weight on this diet to start exercising more, leading them to losing weight even faster. You will feel better, move faster and naturally eat better than you ever have before.

For many of us who have struggled with healthy eating and weight loss, the fasting days have also made us much more aware of what we eat, when we eat and how we eat. It also teaches you that you need to use mealtimes to fuel your body instead of just feeding an appetite. Throughout your course of the 5:2 Diet, you will learn to make healthier meal choices and savor each and every meal, even if it is tiny. Your increased energy and that very special feeling of freedom from cravings, processed foods and all around anxiety will help your realize how unhealthy your relationship to food once was.

The 5:2 Diet isn't going to be a simple solution to fit right into your jeans from high school nor is it a way to lose mass for your next marathon. Instead, it is a lifestyle change that will completely revolutionize your relationship with food and eating. It will make you a better person apart from the food you eat, will make you look better on the outside and feel better on the inside. The 5:2 Diet isn't some fad that you can throw away nor is it a one-size-fits-all plan. It is something that you will need to put your heart and soul into to see the real results.

# FASTING DAYS

Many people seem to have a problem with the fasting days. They spend most of the time thinking about eating, dreaming about eating, and even just staring at foods. However, you should know that you could still eat on the days that you fast. That is the number one rule of fasting days: Never, ever go a day without eating anything. When we are talking about the 5:2 Diet, we are describing days where you will limit your eating, not completely block it off. To be specific, you should eat about a quarter of the food that your body will generally need. On average, the traditional American woman would eat about 500 calories in a day, and a man would eat about 600 calories. However, there are plenty of resources out there that will allow you to figure out your own specific number if you want to get down to ones and tens.

That limit puts you in a place where you either need to get crafty about what you eat or you need to be very meticulous. The truth is that it is probably both. You will be able to eat about three small meals during your fasting days if you are conscious of your calories.

In truth, some people will end up completely fasting save for water when they are doing the 5:2 or 6:1 dieting plan. But that isn't as common nor is it recommended. You should note that fasting is not something that everyone has to or should do. You will be able to find out more below about the specifics of who should and who should not fast.

# SHOULD YOU FAST?

The truth is that the 5:2 Diet is not an option for everyone. For some people, it might be for a mental reason that they shouldn't and for others, it is for a physical reason. Pregnant women should avoid fasting because even after taking away all the nutrition the mother has; the baby will still not get the proper nutrition if the mother does not eat properly. The same thing goes for nursing mothers, it is highly likely that you wouldn't be able to nurse on the days you fast and possible even the day after. Children and teenagers, whose bodies are still changing and growing shouldn't do fasting day either. Most importantly, people who have histories of eating disorders, specifically bulimia or anorexia, should also not participate in a diet that encourages them to fast or they may relapse into old behaviors.

Finally, anyone who has a Type 1 diabetes or Type 2 diabetes should talk to his doctor before taking part in the 5:2 Diet. The same can be said about anyone who is suffering from any acute medical condition or celiac disease. If you have any hesitation at all about participating in the 5:2 Diet, you should ask your doctor before moving any further. They will be able to give you a better idea on how your body and daily life will be impacted by the diet and specifically by the fasting days.

# WHAT YOU CAN EAT

The question always seems to fixate around what you can and what you absolutely cannot eat on your fast days. In theory or at least in a perfect world, you would be able to have whatever you would like – so long as it stays under your daily calorie limit of about 500 or 600 calories.

But the problem with fasting days or at least its first few days isn't really on keeping your planned meals to less than 500 calories. The trouble actually falls when you try to keep those pesky hunger pangs at bay. Those pangs are what make you binge on pretzels, chips, and ice cream right before you go to bed – giving your poor digestion, bad dreams and completely ruining your fasting day. That is why it makes the most sense to eat as smart as you possibly can on your fasting days. Instead of filling your quota in one meal, focus instead on the foods that are naturally filling but that don't have too many empty calories. Those foods will keep you fuller for longer and will also leave you feeling like you actually ate. A square of a candy bar has the same amount of calories as quite a few cups of lettuce. Among the 2, what do you think is the most filling? Instead of eating cheap or processed foods with empty calories, choose something with a high fiber content like:

Generous portions of vegetables, especially leafy green vegetables like kale and spinach

Smaller portions of lean meats like chicken, fish such as salmon or eggs. Bake or roast rather than fry your foods – and do not even think about breading. If you need extra flavor, try blackened.

Soups are a great option for your lower calorie days as they are

7

extremely hearty and warming. Make sure you choose a broth-based soup and not a cream-based soup – surely what you will get would be far more filling.

In the summertime, try to make salads that are dressed with vinegar and herbs instead of creamy dressings like ranch or creamy Italian.

You can (and should, in any diet plan) drink plenty of fresh water. You can mix fresh water with berries, lemons or cucumbers. But remember to add those to your calorie count if you actually consume them.

You can also drink things like black coffee or tea (milk or cream will add unnecessary calories), herb teas and diet drinks, although artificially sweetened drinks may still affect your blood sugar or insulin levels which is not ideal on a fast/restricted day.

If you absolutely have to take milk in hot drinks, remember to include the calories in your allowance.

# WHAT YOU SHOULD AVOID

Remember what we said: "In a perfect world, you will be able to eat whatever you want." Well, you can eat what you want, but in minimal for some food so that you would be able to get the best possible results on your diet. You would want to avoid large-scale portions of those deadly processed carbohydrates – white bread, pasta, cereals, and rice – on your Fasting Days. You may also want to cut out sugary foods and most fruits – berries are the best bet if you want something sweet to eat or if you are craving things that are sweet.

# HOW OFTEN YOU SHOULD EAT

On your fasting days, you will be able to eat up to three times (meals) per day though the meals will all be quite smaller than you are used to eating. Some evidence suggests that the health benefits may be greater if you stick to one or two meals at a higher calorie level than three meals at a smaller calorie count. One big meal that takes up all of your calories is not recommended either. How you spend those two meals really depends on you, your family, your preferences and your own stomach and hunger pangs. You can eat in any combination: breakfast and lunch; lunch and dinner; breakfast and dinner. Most people tend to skip breakfast because they can have a cup of coffee and that will hold them over. Other people find it easier to skip lunch because they are working and not thinking about their hunger pangs. We do not recommend skipping dinner because it will leave you famished and wake you up during the night.

# WHEN YOU SHOULD FAST

Another common question that many people have about their fasting days is when exactly should they schedule them - meaning what days of the week should they choose to fast. Most people will find that it is much easier to split the fasting days up so that they wouldn't go hungry for two straight days especially if being hungry impacts their general mood. Most people choose to fast on a Tuesday and Thursday. Mondays usually do not work because some people consider it as the worst day of the week. Fridays are usually out of the question too since people usually go out on Friday nights. Weekends aren't regarded as good times either because people would like to relax and enjoy on those days.

Whatever days of the week you choose, make sure that they are a day apart because the hunger pains and that grazing feeling can be stronger. A two-day fast can be tougher when you are just starting the diet. Of course, if it isn't possible to do it any other day of the week, then going two days in a row is better than skipping.

It is better for your lifestyle or schedule to do a "back to back" fast if you've already been dieting for a long time. Just don't exceed 48 hours in a row or you can go into that starvation mode that we talked about. Also, don't forget you can pick different days to fast to better suit your plans each week – nothing here is set in stone!

Sample Meal Plans:

## Meal Plan #1

Breakfast: Muller Light Strawberry yogurt (89 calories) mixed with 25 blueberries (20cals). Daily total so far = 109.

Lunch: Weight Watchers approved Tomato Soup (76 calories) and two smaller rice cakes or quinoa cakes (70 calories). Daily total so far = 255.

Dinner: Low-fat spiced lamb skewers come in at 239cals. Total intake for the whole day = 494 calories.

## Meal Plan #2

Breakfast: Make yourself a fruit salad of 1 banana (90 calories), 25 blueberries (20 calories), and a kiwi (46 calories). Daily total so far = 156.

Lunch: Try Young's Cod Steak in Parsley Sauce (101 calories.) To make it even more filling, eat it on a big bed of lettuce (4 calories). Daily total so far = 261.

Dinner: Try any recipe that makes a veggie Balti. (Our recipe is 211 calories). Total intake for the whole day = 494 calories.

# HOW HEALTHY IS THE 5:2 DIET?

Many people question how healthy the 5:2 Diet or any diet that includes intermittent fasting really can be. Once again, the diet is absolutely not healthy for that small group of people that we previously mentioned. For everyone else, the diet is perfectly healthy and even recommended.

Cutting back on your calories two days a week is not harmful to you. In fact, can help train you and your body to accept the things that are better for you. It gives your body a chance to repair some of the internal damages, sequester the inflammation and actually use all of the food that you have already eaten. Remember, even if you are starting to feel uncomfortable or light headed, a lot of it is actually in your head. Our ancient ancestors evolved to thrive on patterns of fasting and feasting – and we can too if we just train our bodies to get back into the swing of things.

This diet will stop your addiction to foods that are bad for you. Research has shown that our bodies are addicted to things that are actually bad for us. Things like wheat (gluten), dairy, sugar and even the chemicals used to process our foods. You will focus more on eating whole foods and the things that will give you energy throughout the day. The 5:2 Diet is something that, eventually, you may even be able to successfully leave without gaining all of the weight you lost back again. You will learn the importance of eating within your limits and eating the good foods that will fill you up. Surprisingly, you will start to crave those good foods like kale, spinach, chicken, salmon, and even some seafood options.

Current research, by professional nutritionists and those who care about how dieting and how we eat affects the body, on intermittent fasting – the broad, general term for diets that use fasting days like 5:2 – suggests that the approach is at least as effective as, if not more effective than, 'normal' dieting where you cut calories by a certain percentage every day. Further research is investigating some of the potential benefits to intermittent dieting in terms of blood sugar and the 'inflammatory response' in the body that is a factor in many medical conditions, including cardiovascular disease, cancer and dementia.

Overall, how healthy is this diet or any other diet, actually depends on your current health status. How quickly you put your body into the diet and the foods that you eat on your diet. If you have questions, you should contact your primary care physician and also consider hiring a nutritionist. If you are really serious or you go to a gym, you might want to talk to one of the trainers about what he or she eats on a daily basis to get an idea on food intake.

If you feel like the diet isn't working for you or is making you sick, contact your doctor and set the record straight. You can also play around with your fasting days, cut it down to one day a week to start with or just change around how many calories you eat and slowly whittle them down to 500 as the weeks pass by you. Part of this diet is learning how to read your body and what is it telling you: Learn to understand it; you do not need a translator.

# FEELING HUNGRY ON THE 5:2 DIET

On any diet and sometimes even when you aren't on an active diet, you will feel hungry. You will feel even hungrier on those fasting days where you do not eat as much as you usually do. You are more likely to feel those hunger pains on the first few days or weeks that you are on the diet. In reality, a lot of those hunger pains actually come from your head. You are aware that you are eating less, so you think that you should be hungry. However, as time passes, you will learn some ways to control your hunger or you just won't be as hungry anymore. Overtime, you'll probably be surprised at how quickly any pain passes, especially if you are kept busy with work or other activities. Those hunger pains won't be something you will have to deal with on a daily or even weekly basis. They are most common on the first few fasts that you do and also on the first fast of the week. Some people do report that they feel colder or experience headaches – both of these are common with all diets. Some people will also experience mood swings or anger. Most people find it getting easier after the first one of the two fasts.

Like what we have said before, the intermittent fasting diet is generally safe for most healthy people, but on the first few fast days, it's worth keeping a small snack handy in case you do feel unwell or dizzy. If you do feel like fainting – which is very rare on this particular diet plan– then don't hesitate to eat something with substance and talk to your doctor before trying out the same diet again.

Afraid of your hunger pangs? Here are some ways to quell them without eating:

## Eat breakfast if they are really bad, even on fasting days

Skipping breakfast, while you are fasting, can generate stomach hunger pains that will also lead to snacking and binging later in the day, and therefore completely ruining your fasting day. If you are experiencing hunger pains at a specific time of day, you may need to change around the meals that you eat during the day. Hunger pains generally begin anywhere from 12 to 24 hours after the last time you ate food, so if you have not gone that long, it might just be in your head. Take note that these pains are usually a lot more intense in younger people (18-34) because they have more "muscle tone" than older people.

## Keep hydrated

Many people have heard the idea of drinking eight glasses of water a day. While that exact number is debated, the right answer is that you should drink a lot of water in a day – some people project the number to be closer to 3 liters of water for women. Many people tend to confuse hunger pangs with being thirsty. If you are feeling hunger pains, take a big drink and see how you feel.

## Add some spices to your daily meals or snacks

Spicy foods are some of the biggest secrets inside of the dieting industry. People think many add them to create taste, and while spices do that, they also keep you fuller for longer. You can control your hunger pangs by sending "full" messages to the brain. Fill your foods with spicy aromas like ginger, turmeric, curry, chili powder, and cayenne. You can add these to things like chicken, soups, and even chips. Try mixing them up and make kale chips, which are low calorie and filling. These plant extracts also increase metabolism, which will help you to see an improvement in weight loss.

## Eat protein every four hours (within the diet)

Lean proteins can act as an appetite suppressant, working within your body to help control hunger pangs and that hungry feeling. Eating just two to three ounces of protein with your meal will trigger a 25 percent spike in energy, allowing you to go work out or continue through your day without the need for sugary drinks that are laden with fat. This will also increase fat metabolism by about 32 percent. Protein also keeps your metabolism at a higher level for about four hours after you eat it. Remember that protein is not found only in meats but in some grains and dairy products like Greek yogurt.

### Watch how much sugar you eat

Sugar, though certainly delicious, is also fake filler – you might feel full now, but about twenty minutes from now, you will feel better. And it isn't just those foods that say "sugar" on the side. Sugar comes in many different names and faces like corn syrup, high-fructose corn syrup, brown sugar, honey, maltose, corn sweeteners and dextrose. You don't want to eat foods that have simple sugars alone in the meal. You will want to mix up what you eat so that you get the full effect of what you are eating. Remember that the brain is extremely sensitive and corn syrup actually confuses it to the point where it does not know if it is full or if it is still hungry. Usually, if it has to choose, it will choose to feel hungry.

### Exercise regularly

Exercising and using up the calories that you are consuming will actually help you feel hungry longer into the day. This might seem counteractive, but you actually run on endorphins after an exercise that chases away many of the other feelings that you may have, including hunger and pain.

### Become a smart snacker

Many people fail on their diets because they snack too much and don't realize the sheer amount of food that they are eating. You should keep your snack on non-fasting days to about 100 calories or less on a regular daily calorie goal. If you have to snack, try to eat things that are healthier and will work to reduce hunger pangs like fruits, vegetables, nuts and seeds and low-fat dairy products.

### Slow down when you eat

Americans tend to eat way too quickly when they do sit down to have a meal. Eating slowly will help you to feel fuller and will reduce the risk of hunger pains. Eating slowly will also cause you to consume fewer calories when you do eat because your brain will recognize that you are hungry for a longer time.

### Make the chewing motion with your jaws

Chewing things like low-calorie gum which simulates the movement of eating, will help to stop them in their tracks when you feel stomach hunger coming on.

## Stomach pains may be unrelated to hunger

If you have tried all of these methods and you still feel those hunger pains, then you may have a problem that is not related to your dieting plan. The pain may be caused by some gastrointestinal disorder that is in the early stages and such disorders can be isolated and treated if caught early.

# HOW DO I EAT ON NORMAL DAYS?

Eating on your "normal days" means that you need to take advantage of your meals and fill up on the things that will carry you through your fasting days. However, in the world we live in today, many people don't know what a "normal" meal actually looks like – our portions are blown way up in size and we think we are cutting calories when we are actually just eating a normal amount. Here's how to eat on your normal days:

**Breakfast:**

Breakfast serves to kick-start your metabolism and gets your body ready to start the day. You should definitely include some lean protein at breakfast and make sure to put some eggs, salmon, lean ham, or low-fat dairy on your plate right away. You will actually burn more calories digesting protein than you would when you are digesting carbs, so even though you really want to eat only toast, it isn't in your best option. Plus you have to think about how much you will be revving up your metabolism, giving yourself a leg up on the day and because foods that are higher in protein will keep you fuller for longer, you will most likely be able to eat fewer calories the rest of the day, and you won't have those hunger pains that we just talked about.

A protein breakfast does not have to be some complicated affair that takes a long time to prepare. You can simply top your morning toast, muffin, or bagel with some scrambled eggs (yolk included), smoked salmon, lean ham, or even with nuts that have high amounts of protein. There are many choices so you will be able to change it up every day.

Whatever you do, on the days when you are not skipping meals to fit into your fasting calories, do not skip breakfast on your normal days, as this will actually set your blood sugar into a complete frenzy, which means that you will end up binging or looking for foods that are bad for you later in the day. Even if it means getting up a few minutes earlier that day, remember that breakfast makes one of the most important parts of your day and helps to count towards your daily intake. That wives' tale is true; eating a good breakfast can help you to keep a level weight.

**Snack:**

Eating a little snack in the middle of the morning, around 9 or 10, is the ideal way to manage your blood sugar levels and to stop yourself from eating something you don't really need. You are less likely to make poor choices if you plan your meals ahead of time. Just make sure that every snack you have will count as a healthy meal and choose from nourishing options that supply you with both the 'pick me up' you need while fitting into your nutritional plan.

Consider having premeasured almonds (so you don't accidentally eat the whole can) or hummus and vegetables.

**Lunch:**

Make yourself a nice, big lunch that is low in calories with a mixture of lean protein and starchy carbohydrates that will keep you full throughout the rest of your workday. Carb-rich foods, though they tend to get a bad reputation, actually supply you with tons of energy. Without them, you will suffer from that classic mid-afternoon slump that causes you to be really moody or causes you to go home and meet up with your pals Ben and Jerry. The key in eating carbohydrates effectively is to choose from the carbs that will produce a steady rise in blood sugar. That means that those packaged baked goods or any of those the sugary 'white' foods are not going to be what you want to eat. Instead, you should be going for the high fiber whole-grains in healthy carbs, which will help you to manage those afternoon munchies and stay in a good mood.

If you do have a sweet tooth, satisfy those cravings and the need for energy with pieces of fresh or dried fruit. Partaking in just a small handful of some dried fruit that has been combined with unsalted nuts or seeds provide you with both the protein and healthy fats that you need to keep you satisfied till supper.

### Dinner:

You can still have carbs at dinner, even if you eat a little later than you normally would. Carbs, at least those healthy ones, are low in fat, high in fiber, and will help you to relax and sleep well at night. Don't eat them alone, however, but combine those carbs with other types of foods, like some healthy essential fats. Look for the ones you find in oily fish like salmon, mackerel, and sardines as well as nuts, seeds, and their oils. Your body will be able to use these healthy fats while you are sleeping for regeneration and repair, which is important for maintaining healthy skin and hair.

# EXERCISING AND MOVEMENT

Another popular question that many people ask about the 5:2 Diet is whether or not you can exercise during the diet, and specifically whether or not you can exercise on the days that you are fasting. The answer is an emphatic YES! Keep exercising like you normally would.

You might not want to go as hard as you normally do when you are first starting to fast because you may get very dizzy. You should always keep some extra food with you and know how to listen to your body. If it tells you to slow down, then you need to slow down and maybe sit on the bike instead of running on the elliptical.

Listen to your body and know when to stop.

If you have any questions, you will need to know when and how to ask your doctor about them. With any diet that restrict calories, your body will go into repair mode because it does not have as many calories to burn as it normally would. This makes it so that you have much, much less energy for your body to use. If you put in too much effort, you may feel faint or you might even feel like you are going to throw up. We recommend checking with a doctor, especially if you have any previous heart problems and get your blood pressure checked to ensure you are able to work out while on this diet.

In the end, many of us do exercise while fasting with no ill effects. It may be a good idea to avoid very vigorous exercise until after your first couple of fasts – and if you feel unwell, listen to your body and stop.

Make sure that when you exercise, you are fully hydrated and eat one of your small meals before you run. You might want to take this day to do something like yoga, stretching, or floor exercises. Using equipment or machines can result in you hurting yourself if you do pass out.

One thing that you can note about exercising while on the 5:2 Diet is that you shouldn't add any additional calories burned through exercise to your calorie allowance on a fast day – stick to 500-600 calories a day.

# WEIGHT LOSS

People on the 5:2 diet have lost varying amounts of weight: from those who simply maintained their weight to those who have lost over 100 pounds by sticking to the diet for a longer amount of time.

If you want to track your weight loss, weigh yourself before you start the dieting plan. You may also want to get some measurements and chart your BMI. Pick a day of the week and take all of those measurements every day to see how your body changes. You can find apps or online programs that will allow you track the changes – seeing them in a chart will make you want to do more and push harder. Remember that the rate at which you will lose weight depends on many things: age, gender, activity level, body, history, food choices, and exercise levels. Weight loss is usually much faster in the beginning and once your body gets used to the idea, you tend to lose weight at a slower level. That is when some people add in a third day of fasting.

Weight loss is much faster for those people who have a significant amount of weight to lose. For those who are trying to reach a healthy weight from a very unhealthy weight, you need to remember that as you lose weight, the amount of weight you lose each and every week will go down, so don't feel discouraged. The important thing to remember about the 5:2 Diet is that it's very sustainable – and you're more likely to be able to maintain the loss.

You should also remember that weight loss fluctuates based on the time of the week. That is why we suggested weighing yourself only once a week. Things like hormones, digestion and even phases of the moon can affect your weight by quite a few pounds. Things like water and bloating can also add to your weight. Remember that if you are building muscles, you might even gain a few pounds because muscles weigh more than fats.

There might be some trouble if you go past three or four weeks without losing any weight. IN that case, you might want to try some of these – especially if you have not strayed from your dieting and exercise plans:

Take before and after selfies that will allow you to see if your body is changing. Keep the same clothes so that you can really compare what is happening in the picture and just how the clothes feel.

Buy or find a piece of clothing that was tight at the beginning of the diet or that is currently tight. Then, try that piece of clothing on every week. Some women use their prom dresses or jeans from when they were in high school. No matter what you choose, by using the clothing method, you'll often notice changes that aren't yet showing on the scales.

Calculate something called the TDEE or Total Energy Expenditure. There are many apps that will allow you to figure it out on your own without the help of a doctor. This will be a rough estimate of how many calories you can eat each day to maintain your weight – which you can then use to get your personalized 5:2 fasting days total.

Add up the amount of calories that you consume on a typical or normal day to make sure you're not over-doing it with the diet or the cutting of food. Of course remember that our consumption will vary naturally day to day, but it's a useful guideline.

Equally, some people find if they're under-eating by a lot on normal days, it can affect weight loss due to changes within the body. So try to adopt sensible, sustainable eating patterns.

No matter what, remember that when you lose weight at a slower rate, you will far be more likely to keep that weight off. Remember that putting weight back on is a lot easier than you think it might be – so eat up and eat well, but don't forget to exercise in addition to your diet if you want the best weight loss chances.

# IS THE 5:2 A LIFESTYLE CHANGE?

This has a simple answer, and a complicated one. Yes, you will be changing your lifestyle. You will have to change everything from what you buy to how you cook the foods that you want to eat. You will be changing your life, as you know it.

But there are also so many great changes that come from adapting your life to the 5:2 Diet. You will be more mindful about what you eat, how you eat, and when you eat. You will have a better relationship with foods. You will have the chance to see how your diet affects how you feel, how you act, and what you can accomplish.

5:2 isn't as much of a diet as it is a lifestyle change. You won't need to mix in new things, but you will just change how you eat two days a week. Sure, it may result in you taking away calories from your daily life, but that does not mean that you have to start eliminating the things you love. This is all about moderation and eating the things that you love, but either changing them so that they are healthier or eating them only on special occasions.

So yes, this is a lifestyle changer. But in reality, it is so much more than that as well. It is simply a life changer – your life will never be the same after you learn these tips and tricks. You will never be able to look at food the same way again and that is definitely not a bad thing.

# CONCLUSION

Many of us that have come to know and love this dieting plan actually hope to stay on 5:2 for life because it feels so easy and natural to us. We have been doing it for years and it is now something that is second nature. We don't think of it as a diet anymore, it is simply a new way to look at things. That's not to say that we don't go out and enjoy ourselves because we do. We have just changed the way we live on a normal day – we still eat birthday cakes, Thanksgiving stuffing, and summer ice cream.

Moderation – it's the name of the game.

If you stick with the 5:2 Diet, you will be able to reach a healthy weight. Then, you will be able to make some changes. You might like to shift from 5:2 to 6:1 – again, it's your decision, it's your body, and it is your health. Certainly, the health benefits mean it's a plan and a lifestyle that can offer you more than just some weight loss alone.

Good luck on your mission to be happier and healthier in your life. You will find that you will easily slip into this diet and that you can start whenever you want. You can pick tomorrow, you can wait until Monday, or you can wait until the start of the next month. Whatever you choose, go into this with an open mind. Don't rush yourself, give yourself encouragement, find a buddy, and never give up hope that you can get to where you want to be, just as long as you trust yourself.

Finally, if you enjoyed this book, please click below to share your thoughts and post a positive review on Amazon. I would greatly appreciate your support! If you feel you did not receive value from reading this book, please email bookguarantee@plaid-enterprises.com for instructions to receive a refund - no hard feelings.

Thank you and good luck!

Kara Aimer

GRAB YOUR FREE REPORT HERE - LOSE 10LB IN 7 DAYS!
http://www.plaid-enterprises.com/52

Visit Kara Aimer Online and Get Your FREE Book:
http://www.plaid-enterprises.com/kara-aimer

www.ingramcontent.com/pod-product-compliance
Lightning Source LLC
Chambersburg PA
CBHW070525290526
45790CB00003B/1295